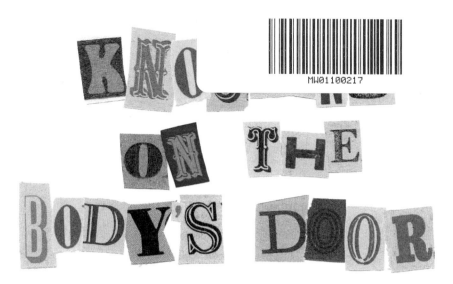

KNOCKING ON THE BODY'S DOOR

Poems to Read on the
Bathroom Floor

By Sita Gaia

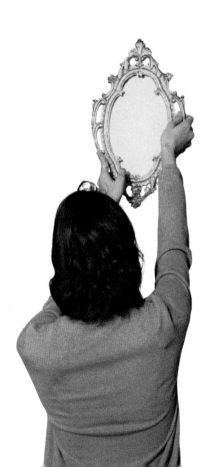

Knocking on the Body's Door is a lighthouse for anyone who's ever felt alone in their suffering. Sita Gaia asks 'what does isolation feel like on your skin?' and then answers by finding hope and community even in her own darkness. Their poems are an honest window into the life of someone living with chronic illness and allow the reader to feel empathy for 'how the body shrinks into less of a person'. It made me rethink how much I take for granted and left me grateful that Sita gives a voice to something not yet widely spoken about. These poems bring truth and comfort equally and will leave you changed for the better.

- Melissa Sussens, Runner up: *New Contrast National Poetry Prize*

In Knocking on The Body's Door, Sita Gaia shines a light on what her life with epilepsy is like. How it is more than just a list of symptoms, how it can be the jealous third wheel at a first date, the breath you hold when you pour your tea, Ashton Kutcher in the shower or a door holder for depression. Her words make it tangible. This book will hold me past its last letter.

- Nadine Klassen, published in *Emotional Alchemy*

"...There isn't a healthy body in the world that is stronger than a sick person's spirit."- Andrea Gibson

Dedicated to all the Chronic Illness Warriors.
It's a hard walk, but never, ever give up.

ACKNOWLEDGEMENTS

Thank you to Prolific Pulse Press LLC for taking such careful work with my poems. Thank you to Lisa Joy Tomey for working closely with me throughout the process.

I would also like to thank *Fine Lines Literary Journal* for originally publishing the poem "Terra," *Harness* magazine for publishing "Turning on the Flashlight in the Grey Hallway," and *Last Leaves* Magazine for publishing "Metal Toilet." Thank you to Susan Alexander, thank you to Megan Falley, Melissa Sussens, and Nadine Klassen for your lovely words.

Thank you to my mentors who "taught" me about poetry since I was growing up. Jude Neale, who taught me in Grade 3 that line breaks were essential to poetry. Megan Falley, who taught me to dig around into the deeper meaning of my poems and to "show" not tell.

Further, poets who have inspired me, such as Rupi Kaur, W.H. Auden, Andrea Gibson, Mary Oliver, Sabrina Benaim, and Angel Nafiz.

Further inspired by Bree Bailey, Katie Müeller, Jo Pangolin, Kason Seward, BA Powers, Jason Terry, Kika Man and Melissa Sussens. You have been my rocks.

I would like to thank every member of *Poems That Don't Suck*, and Megan Falley for creating such a rich writing community. Each member has given me the courage to see what is possible. This book would not be here without your support. I would also like to thank my Terra, for being as excited as I am, and continuously being there for me. Mum, Dad, Jules and kk, thank you for celebrating my wins along with me. Also, a huge thank you goes out to Johanna Bartels for doing the cover art and inside art.

TABLE OF CONTENTS

Terra

Her eyes look at me serenely
the most beautiful green you would ever see.
Compliments seem to the thing of the hour
I look away, bashful,

while she is amused by my shyness,
she knows me as the confident girl
who asks her out on the first date
not just to chill-but an actual date.

A seizure wants to join us on the date though,
 it is inconsiderate in that way
cutting the bottom of my chin open.

The universe works in funny ways,
 as she has enough Kleenex from Bronchitis a month prior.
She joins me on the ground hoping to comfort me.

In my seizure state I pull her arms around me,
a hug during a traumatic moment.
My unconscious brain knows how to woo what it wants.

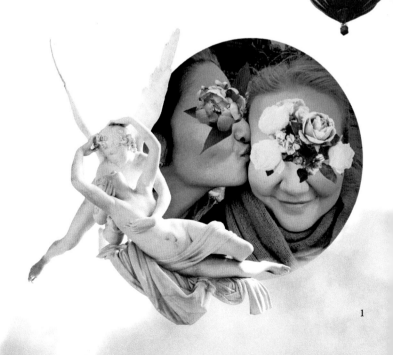

1

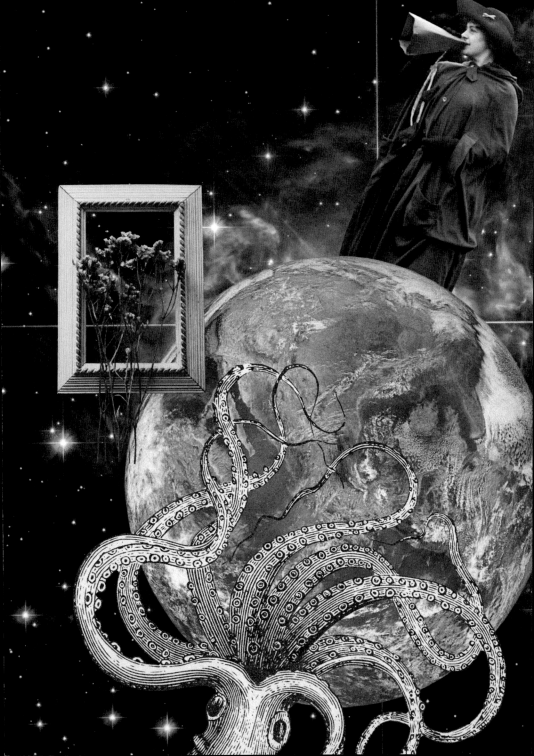

Things About My Chronic Illness You Should know

1. I hate pity. I didn't ask to have an illness, and your pity only makes it worse.

2. I am not lucky I cannot work full time because of my illness. In my best life, I am working 40 hours a week, and still able to go to the gym after work.

3. I hate resting after an episode. Most people with chronic illnesses would agree that it sucks to miss out due to a flare, an episode, or any other issue with their body they have no control over.

4. Ableist folks drive me mad. When I am fired from my job for disclosing that I have epilepsy, it means that the Manager would rather not have me as a liability.

5. Please don't be amazed by my condition. Sixty-five million people in the world have it too, and I am not alone on this journey.

6. Do not ask me all the places I have had seizures. I have had them everywhere.

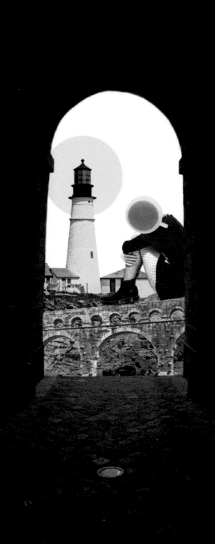

Turning on The Flashlight in The Gray Hallway

Alone on my path of sickness,
friends, over cups of coffee, were so sorry,
but did they know what it was like to hallucinate
Ashton Kutcher in the shower?

Did they know the rainbow of illness
the colors cast on their floor, dim and grey?

Grief is an endless crumbled hallway.
Laughter an echo in my stomach.
My friends don't hold their breath

when they pour a cup of tea.
Once, I forgot to hold mine,
and the kitchen floor was the coldest place

to soothe my burnt body.
Five months of bandages, the truth
under my robe as everyone said *Congratulations!*

and not, *How are you feeling?*
But one day I found a bridge
that fit into my back pocket, a community
who turned on the light in my hallway.

Strange names
with Polaroid photos
I could not
place.

Who also knew the fork of Topamax
topped high with food,
which tasted like nothing
going down.

They knew
what it's like to not know
your own name
after an episode. How the body shrinks into less

of a person. My university professor saying: *Oh
you look so good!* The invalidation of sickness—
Was my body even bad before?
They knew that being too thin was also a sign of sickness.

Their stories on display like an art gallery,
in tiny medicine cups, something
I could finally recognize.
They understood the confusion

of a sudden slumber at work, a fatigue
that hides behind your eyelids, & calls it home.
They knew the embarrassment of an unexpected
crash at the party of Zumba class, breaking

a lamp in the studio, because your brain
had a different agenda than your feet.
My friend in London struggles to make enough
money. I understand. Without my wife, I swim

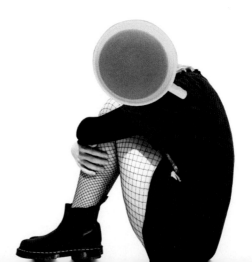

below the poverty level. I tell my friend
across the pond about the polite emails
which exclaim my fingers didn't spin
fast enough to work at the coffee shop.

My avatar texts two purple hearts, the color of epilepsy,
to say, *Together, we are strong like Bulls.*
Drool drips on to my chin while looking
at the recipes my pal with Crohn's posted.

Their phone dings with two growls
from my hungry stomach.
Two orange hearts to those with Multiple Sclerosis.
One friend stuck in bed for 11 weeks.

Sometimes that's all you can do.

You don't know the struggle, don't know
what to say. But know the heart said it all.

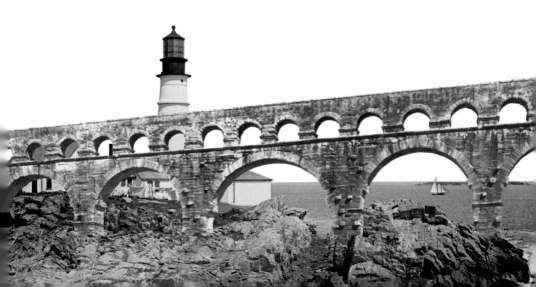

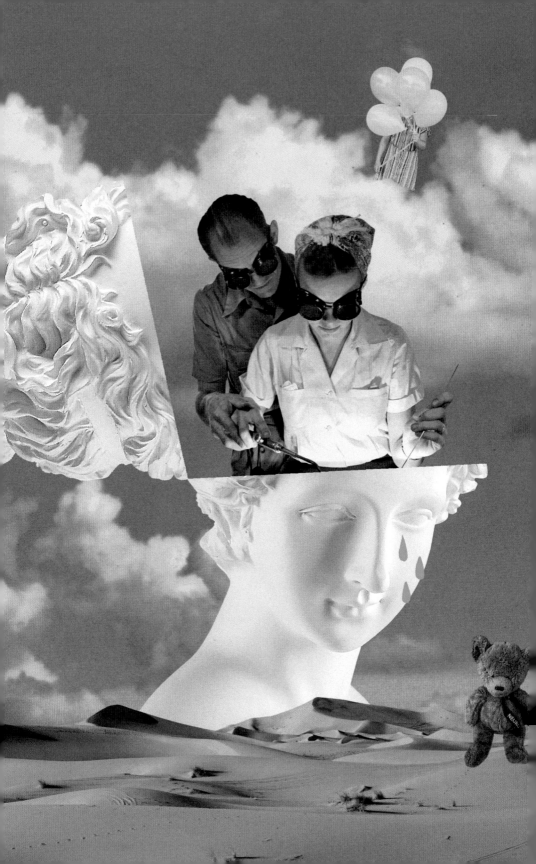

Brain Surgery

For my first appointment with a neurosurgeon,
I wore my favorite clothes and new shoes.
When he said he wanted to insert tiny wires
into my brain with a robotic hand,
I fell for him as hard as my body hit the pavement.

I still remember Genevieve; I needed to arrive freshly
washed for the day of the surgery.
I kept her number in my pocket like a treasure.
I guess it was naive of me to assume they would fix my life.

Too fast I learned that brain surgery involved
four days of puking,
lifting my head for a single moment,
only to wish my Mom a happy birthday.

Some days covered me like a mouldy blanket.
My favourite nurse asked me *what was wrong?*
Not able to point in any specific direction,
he covered my teddy's head in toilet paper and medical tape.

When the wires were taken out
after two weeks, I moved clumps
of hair away from the drain
with my foot.

After finally being cleaned up,
my head neurologist pulled a chair up
to my bed.

My tests yielded zero results.

He may as well have taken my brain right there.
To him, it was fascinating;
while I'd rather trade it in a game
of swapping Christmas gifts.

Hibernation

My body darts around the
the concept of being
well
and being ill.
Like a hummingbird,
I flap my wings ten to fifteen times
per second,
in one place
before you can catch a glance.
When I'm tired, my fatigue
rests into
hibernation.

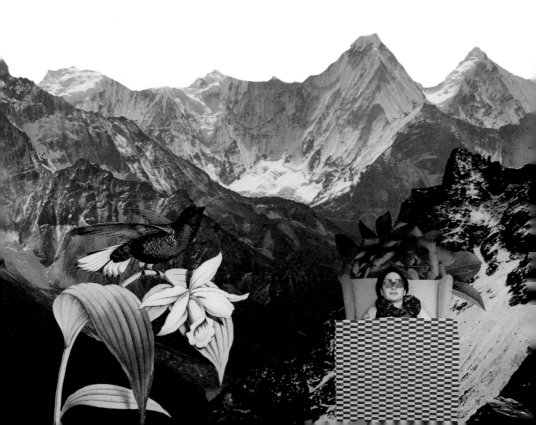

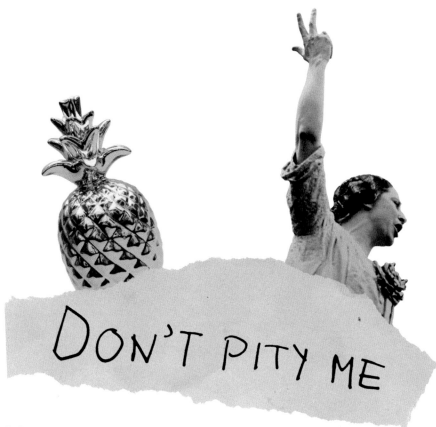

Moxie

Don't pity me
is written with a sharpie
all over
this disabled body,

that's where moxie is from.
Disability is not a shameful thing.
Could it be that it's a reality that people accept?
Sometimes dire—hurting in the gut,

festering wasps in the mind.
Stings so powerful, yet still
don't mess with me.

Girl, you have character.
Don't let it crash and burn.
Grab the cards from the dealer,
& turn them into fucking gold.

Undiagnosed Illness in the Year of 2020

After dealing with
the aftermath,
I summoned

my legs
to be
strong.

Solely to transport
my vessel
to the
washroom.

I spent eleven hours
in the hospital.

Alone.

Burning through my data
as fast as that
one time

Faith and I
shared
a joint.

Doctors said
maybe it's MS or a stroke.
I knew it wasn't.

While doctor's opinions
are strong,
they can be
weak,

like a prescription
scribble. The patient knows
their body the best.

Fumbling out of the
hospital like
a drunk,

my wife in the waiting
room in her pj's,
starting to look

as desperate
as those unemployed
due to COVID-19.

I feebly gripped
my cane like
an old woman

into Dr. A.K.'s office.
He shone a light
into my eye
& said to my mom,
See that? It's toxicity.

Her eye is quivering.

Thank god. Someone knew.

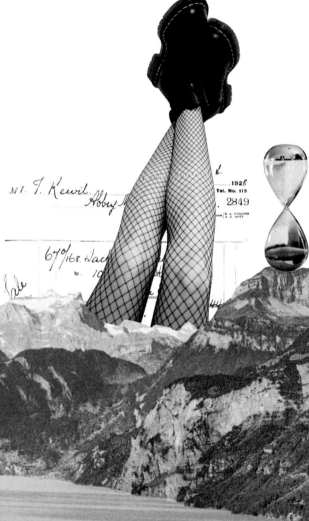

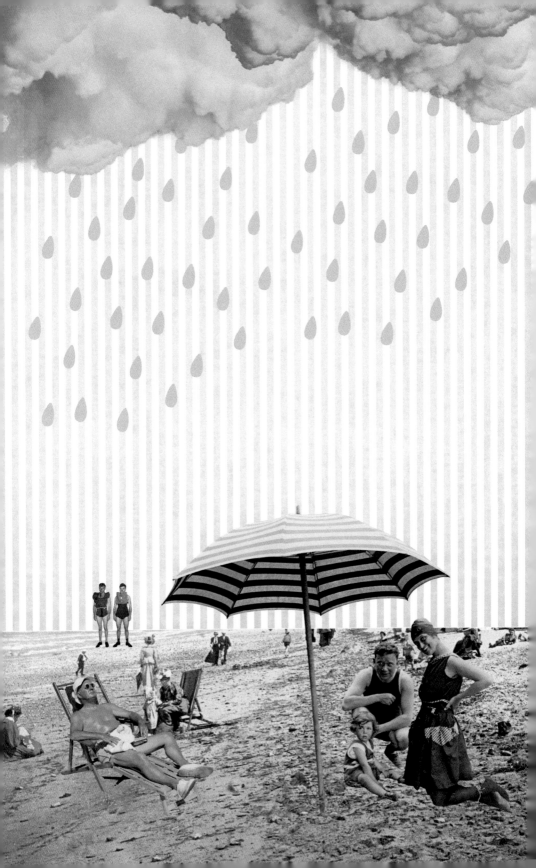

Downpour

I think everyone with
a chronic illness should
have more pyjamas
than daytime clothes.

What does isolation feel like
on your skin?
Is it cold underneath your PJ's?
Or naked and lonely,

waiting for someone
to warm your shivers away
on a sunny California day?
Can you hear your rapid spit fire

thoughts, going off one by one
like an automatic ball
shot out, in your face they say.
They are so messy, you swing

but miss them all.
Or is your brain slow like
he long drag of a hallway
with no end in sight?

Does it continue like a
summer downpour?
The sudden darkness flicking
off the light, holding you

in its isolated embrace.

Metal Toilet

When I told my therapist
my life was better off
in pieces of ash,

he marched me out to my Dad's
car with strict instructions
to go to the emergency immediately.

I fumed like the exhaust
of the tailpipe on my grandpa's car,
before he died an honorable death.

I cavalierly texted
a few friends
about the attempt.

It was not for attention.
I had the perfect opportunity
the night before.

Smothered in love by parents
who were always home,
there was no good time.

Deemed unsafe in my own hands, I
spent the night with the lonely hours
of the clock.

When I used the
washroom,
I found the toilet was metal.

I kicked it so hard
with my blue Converse
low tops.

It was indestructible and steady
as a rock.
I couldn't even be trusted to use
a normal toilet.

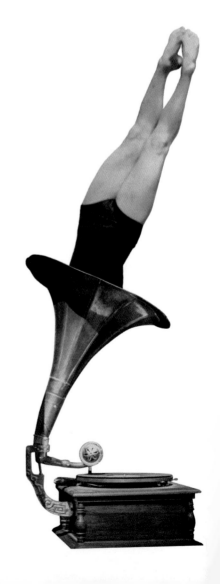

Sometimes it's easier to
shut up about these things.

But that's not what
1-800-SUICIDE
told me.

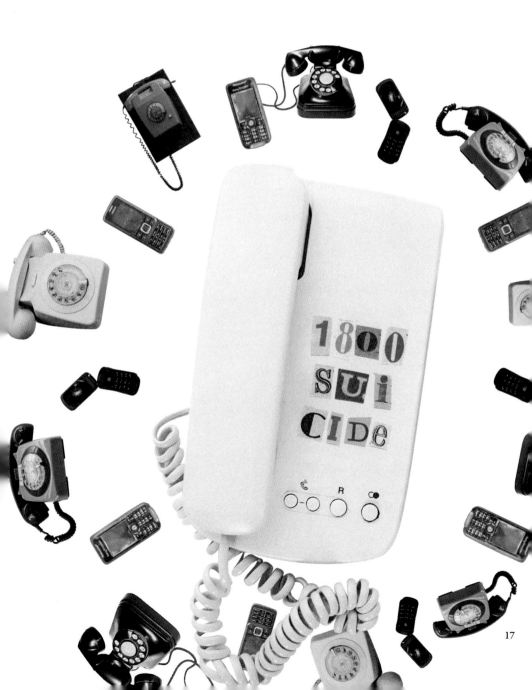

I'll Have a Seizure With my Coffee on the Side

I love the coffee shop down the street.
The grinders,
how people hide behind their laptops
drowning out the world with their headphones- whales
under the sea don't care how far down they are.

The awe of how fast
the baristas punch in my order-
or how some of them have it memorized.
I like consistency.

It amazes me how they
can work while conversation
pours out of me like the coffee
they pour for their patrons.

How they smile at me
because they're friendly,
or just paid to do it,
I don't care.

Did you know that the coffee shop
is the best place
out in the world to have a seizure?
My seizures don't leave me staring
off in one direction.

One time I treated my Mum and I to a coffee,
& I felt the heavy pull
of fatigue from my meds,
collapsed to the ground.

After I 'came to', my mom
wiped up hot coffee from my chest,
using her favourite navy scarf.

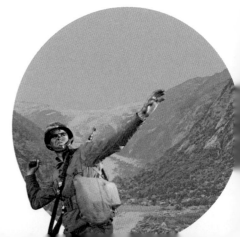

What was my own name?
Where was I and why were people
taking pictures of me?
The smell of coffee
reeked all over my body.

The floor was cold, clean,
but too hard to fall on, right?
Is any floor good to fall on?

No,
I fall without warning
and my head smacks the floor so hard,
I feel my skull move.

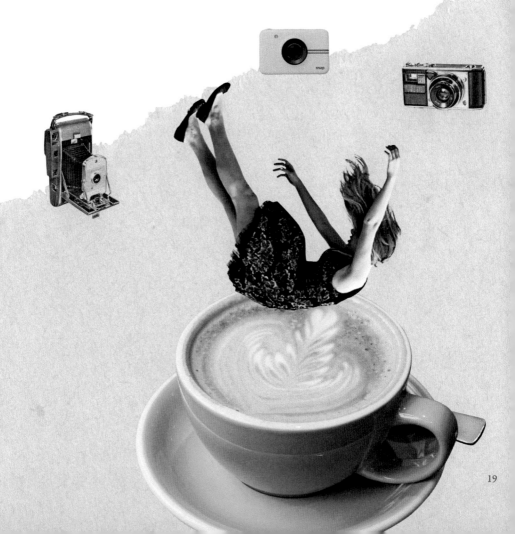

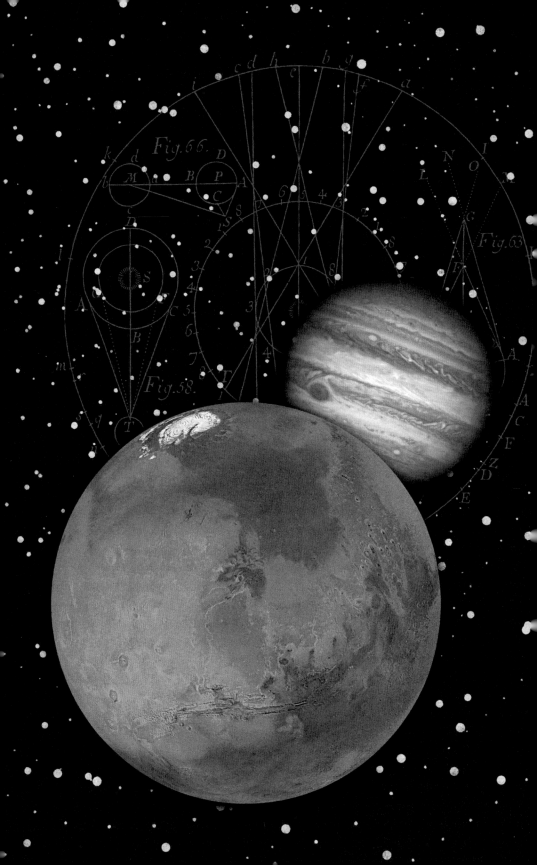

Resiliency

They spoon fed it to me
like it's the first time
Mars and Jupiter met

for the first time in 400 years.
I didn't look that night.
It was one more thing to check off my

to do list, and I was not going
to wait, cold and shivering
to see what the night sky

had on display for me.
Though high in the sky,
I felt its burden tucked around my soul.

Handprints of glitter
smeared across my back,
to show the bright colors

for everyone watching.

My Wife's Thoughts About Poetry

Disgruntled, I wake from a sleep.
My hair is as messy as my wife's
thoughts.
My wife rolls around in the bed,
poems dribbling from her lips.
Someone tell her to work a 9-5,

then I might actually sleep.
3 hours later she traipses in from the bedroom without meter
to wish me good morning.

Morning! It's almost noon!
But we do share the same love for coffee;
her writing is fueled by caffeine and pounding fingers.

A bride to her laptop,
devoted to her screen.
Thank god, I can focus.

I take a quick break
& find a trail of bridal petals on the hardwood floor.
Is she out of her mind?

Her metaphors don't cover
the rent.
My God, can't she help more?
Going cross-eyed staring at spreadsheets,
mundane meetings,
that sometimes last too long

When was the last time I picked up a paint brush?
I could not tell you.
She paces back and forth, almost tripping on her veil.

Let me tell you-her tread is not graceful
I get it from my Mom, she tells me.
All of her repetitions stir anxiety.

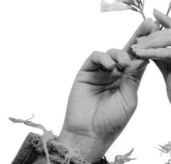

I ask her what she's doing and
does she have to think so close to my desk?
Her thoughts tick back and forth

like a metronome.
I can hear them explode inside her head
like on the first of July,

fireworks light up the sky while dogs huddle under tables.
My deadlines smash me in the face
& I say no, no, no,

no poems on my lunch.
Finally, time is on my side.
I always need his vote.

Crashing to the couch in my comfortable clothes,
business casual is out.
She sits beside me quietly, on the L-shaped
couch of our love.

I scroll through Tik Tok, she is as crumpled
as all the drafts of one poem she's written.
Putting my hand to her back as she cries,
how her peers are so much better
& she's a lousy fraud.

I remind her of reading her poetry at a coveted event
under a tent in the pouring rain.
The youngest poet there.

I may hate poetry,
but don't give up.
Now's not the time.

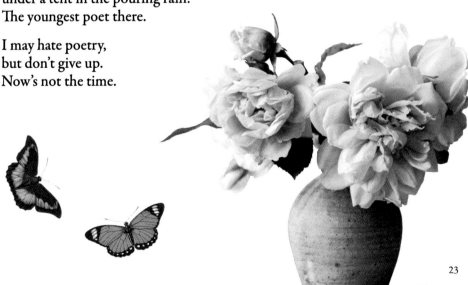

RESOURCES

Epilepsy Resources in Canada

BC EPILEPSY SOCIETY-VANCOUVER & VICTORIA
Phone: 604-875-6704
Email: info@bcepilepsysociety.ca
Web: bcepilepsy.com

EDMONTON EPILEPSY ASSOCIATION
Phone: 740-488-9600
Email: info@edmontonepilepsy.org
Web: edmontonepilepsy.org

EPILEPSY ASSOCIATION OF CALGARY
Phone: 403-358-3358
Program Manager- Louise Gagne: 403-230-2764x105
Web: epilepsycalgary.com

EPILEPSY AND SEIZURE ASSOCIATION OF MANITOBA
Phone: 204-783-0466
email: esam@manitobaepilepsy.org
Web: manitobaepilepsy.org

SASKATCHEWAN EPILEPSY
Phone: 305-359-0905
Email: skepilepsy@sask.tel.net
Web: epilepsysaskatoon.com

EPILEPSY SASKATOON
Phone: 306-665-1939
Email: saskatoon@sasktel.net

EPILEPSY ONTARIO
Phone: 905-738-9431
Email: info@epilepsy.org

EPILEPSY OTTAWA
Phone: 613-594-9255
Web: epilepsyottawa.ca

EPILEPSY TORONTO
Phone: 416-964-9095
Email: info@epilepsytoronto.org
Web: epilepsytoronto.org

ASSOCIATION QUEBECOISE DE L'EPILEPSIE
Contact through their website and click the Contact tab.
Web: associationquebecoiseepilepsie.com/

EPILEPSY MONTREAL METROPOLITAN
Email: h.sauerwein@umontreal.ca

EPILEPSY ASSOCIATION OF THE MARITIMES
Phone: 902-429-2633
Email: ed@epilepsymaritimes.org
Web: epilepsymaritimes.org/

NEWFOUNDLAND AND LABRADOR
Tel: 709-722-0502
E-mail: executivedirector@epilepsynl.com
Web: epilepsynl.com/

NEW BRUNSWICK
Web: 2gnb.ca

❧ Can't find your location?

Check out: canadianepilepsyalliance.org/find-your-local-office/ for more locations.

Mental Health:

CANADIAN MENTAL HEALTH ASSOCIATION, NATIONAL
250 Dundas St. West, Suite 500
Toronto, ON M5T 2Z5
Phone: 416-646-5557
E-mail: info@cmha.ca
Suicide Hotline 24/7: 1-833-456-4566
In QC: 1-866-277-3553
Web: crisisservicescanada.ca

United States Resources

NAEC National Association of Epilepsy Centers
Mental Health:

NATIONAL INSTITUTE OF MENTAL HEALTH
Office of Science Policy, Planning, and Communications
6001 Executive Boulevard, Room 6200, MSC 9663
Bethesda, MD 20892-9663
Email: nimhinfo@nih.gov
Phone: 1-866-615-6464

NATIONAL SUICIDE PREVENTION LIFELINE
Phone 24/7: 800-273-8255

Helpful Books

Gotham Girl Interrupted: My Misadventures in Motherhood, Love, and Epilepsy by Alisa Kennedy Jones

Living Well with Epilepsy and Other Seizure Disorders: An Expert Explains What You Really Need to Know by Carl W. Bazil

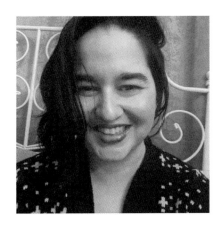

ABOUT THE AUTHOR

Sita Gaia (she/they) is a Social Artist, and a queer chronic illness warrior. She is a TEDx alumnae, and her talk "The Hell of Chronic Illness" has been used across North America in universities as a resource.

She loves Owls and drinks way too much coffee. They have been published through *Poetry Soup*, *Harness Magazine*, *Fine Lines Literary Magazine*, *Last Leaves Magazine* and *Kissing Dynamite magazine*.

They reside in Vancouver, BC with their wife.

You can find them on Instagram at @sitagaia_poetry.

Manufactured by Amazon.ca
Bolton, ON